I0421644

Raw Food Diet:
Detox Diet:

Planted Based Diet & Detox Cleanse Diet to Increase Energy & Natural Weight Loss

Raw Food Diet Guide

Lose Weight Quickly, Achieve Optimal Health and Feel Energized with the Raw Food Diet and Raw Food Recipes

EMMA ROSE

Table of Contents

Introduction

I want to thank you and congratulate you for purchasing the book, *"Raw Food Diet Guide: Lose Weight Quickly, Achieve Optimal Health and Feel Energized with the Raw Food Diet and Raw Food Recipes"*.

This book contains proven steps and strategies on how to effectively apply the raw food diet into your life.

A raw food diet, also known as uncooked diet, is essentially an eating plan that largely involves the consumption of unprocessed and uncooked food. Those who take on this lifestyle are often acknowledged as raw foodists or raw food practitioners. Sometimes, they are referred to as raw food advocates, although this term may also be used to individuals who are interested in or about to convert to the raw food diet.

In the diet, it is believed that cooking or heating of food will destroy the natural enzymes and nutrients typically found in food and produce. This can bring about complications because these enzymes are mainly responsible for fighting off diseases and improving digestion. Therefore, in order to avoid this, raw foodists eat food in its raw state, as the diet's name suggests. This helps alkalize the body, since cooked food has acidic toxins that disrupt the body's acid/alkaline balance. Such disruption often causes illnesses and excess weight. In a nutshell, heating food above 118°F initiates the chemical changes that produce the acidic toxins like free radicals, mutagens and carcinogens, which are normally linked to diseases such as heart problems, arthritis, cancer and diabetes.

There are more than one variations of the diet, and it is entirely up to you how you will shape up your own diet plan. Generally, to be considered a raw foodist, an individual must at least eat 75% to

100% raw, unprocessed and organic food and drink pure water. Most of the items you will eat are plant-based which should never be heated above 115°F. While majority of raw foodists are vegetarian, there are those who opt to consume raw animal products such as raw fish, sashimi, raw milk and the like. Some may also incorporate fresh fruits and vegetables into their meal plan. On the whole, you have the power to create whatever raw food diet structure suits your lifestyle and your preferences best.

Thanks again for purchasing this book, I hope you enjoy it! Please take some time to stop by and LIKE our Facebook page:

https://www.facebook.com/joypublishing

With gratitude,

Emma Rose

Chapter 1

An Overview of the Raw Food Diet

The concept of the raw food diet is simple – cooking diminishes the nutritional value of food. Even though most of the food items in the diet are consumed while it is raw, heating is acceptable provided that the temperature stays between the range of 104 to 118°F or below.

Since cooking is perceived to kill off enzymes naturally found in food, raw food practitioners choose to avoid cooked food. As a matter of fact, overconsumption of cooked food forces the body to work overtime in order to produce more enzymes to support normal bodily functions. In the long run, the lack of enzymes can instigate a lot of problems involving a person's health, particularly accelerated aging, nutrient deficiency, weight gain and digestive problems.

Going raw can prove to be challenging, especially for those that are just starting out. It takes a lot of discipline to stick to the principles of the diet. Moreover, extra effort is required mentally and physically. When it comes to preparing your daily raw meals, your options are limited. Here are some of the procedures you may apply when organizing your meal plan:

- *Germination* – this is the process of soaking in water for a certain period of time. The recommended amount of time differs from one person to another but for raw foodists, the safest bet is to soak overnight.

- *Sprouting* – this comes after germination. After the beans, legumes or seeds are soaked, they may then be sprouted. Items should be left at room temperature until a sprout comes out of it. These sprouts may then be used for preparing food but should be rinsed and drained thoroughly beforehand.

- *Blending* – involves the use of a blender or food processor in order to create sauces, smoothies, or soup among others.

- *Dehydrating* – employs an equipment known as a dehydrator, which simulates sun drying. Common products of dehydrators are crackers, croutons, raisins, fruit leathers, sundried tomatoes, breads and kale chips.

- *Pickling* – a method of preserving food by marinating in a brine.

- *Juicing* – the process of extracting of vitamins, minerals and natural juices from plant tissues, particularly raw fruits and vegetables.

- *Fermentation* – process of converting sugar to carbon dioxide through the use of yeast.

Now that you know what procedures are available to you when preparing your raw meals, the next thing to know is which particular equipment/s you need to use. Below are some of the staple equipment that can be seen in every raw foodist's kitchen:

- *Dehydrator* – it is an enclosed container that has heating elements that can warm at low temperatures. It has a fan that blows warm air onto the food.

- *Spiral Slicer* – slices vegetables into spiral shapes

- *Thermometer* – to ensure that temperature stays below 118°F when heating food.

- *Trays* – for soaking and sprouting beans, legumes or seeds

- *Sprouters* or *mason jars*

- *Food processor*

- *Blender*

- *Juicer*

These are the basic things you have to know if you intend to convert to the raw food diet. Now that you have an idea of what it is and how it works, you will then have to figure out why you would want to choose this lifestyle.

Chapter 2

Why Do People Go Raw?

To some people, converting to a raw food diet seems like a crazy idea. After all, why would anyone want to give up eating all the delectable cooked dishes for uncooked food? How could one survive solely on salads? Why should you limit your choices when eating? These are just some of the many questions people ask when it comes to changing up their diet. Truth be told, there is a less-than-enthusiastic reception from others. Despite these doubts and uncertainties about the diet, those who choose to go raw are very passionate about adhering to the lifestyle. In fact, raw food diet practitioners more often than not retain this routine for years or even for the rest of their lives.

For those who are wondering why someone would stick to such a challenging and demanding way of life, there are several reasons why people take on the diet. For most, optimal health is the primary objective. Some choose to uphold their philosophical and ethical principles. Then there are others who are merely drawn to the diet's environment-friendly quality. These objectives are further explained below.

Health Reasons

Perhaps the most typical reason why anyone would want to begin a raw food diet is the fact that it is beneficial to one's health. For one, it helps prevent and fight off diseases because of the abundance of vitamins, minerals, nutrients and antioxidants that help reduce risks of illnesses or slow down its progress. It also helps that raw food has a lack of calories, saturated fat, cholesterol and other possibly harmful elements normally found in cooked, processed food. Weight loss is also a huge motivation for raw foodists, since a raw diet rich in fiber and low in calories is a great, fast way to shed pounds. Overall, one's health and well-being is positively affected by the raw food diet.

Philosophical and Ethical Reasons

There are a number of individuals who prefer to apply raw food diet because it is in line with their philosophical and ethical beliefs and principles. These are the same people who refuse to purchase animal meat and processed food. As an alternative, these people choose to support organic agriculture and food coming from plants. A moral code like this is surprisingly a strong incentive for some to go raw.

Environmental Reasons

Environmental benefits were once viewed merely as a bonus as opposed to a primary purpose for going raw, particularly for raw vegan foodists. The cooking and processing of food items also have great effect on the environment. Gigantic amounts of resources are used in the food processing industry. Furthermore, most raw foodists encourage organic agriculture, hence using their money to buy food and advocate against the use of chemical fertilizers, herbicides and pesticides that can damage and eventually destroy the environment.

These are the principal reasons why an individual would want to apply the raw food diet and make it a part of his or her daily routine. Raw foodists have their own opinions and motives for considering such a lifestyle choice.

Chapter 3

Raw Food Recipes to Get You Started

This wide array of recipes will help you sustain a raw food diet without getting tired of eating the same food over and over again.

Sauces, Dressings and Condiments

Most meals are dull and boring without sauces and condiments. A delicious sauce can add more taste and flavor to a dish. However, some worry that by following a diet, one must ultimately give up the use of sauces and condiments. While you cannot use the traditional processed sauces, you may create your own using the recipes below.

1. Silica-Rich Dressing

Cucumbers are packed with the minerals responsible for nourishing connective tissues such as the nails, hair, bones and skin. Moreover, they are naturally refreshing and hydrating. By using cucumbers in this recipe, they allow oil reduction, which makes this dressing a low-calorie option.

Ingredients:

- 1 ¼ cups of cucumber, chopped, peeled and seeded
- 2 tablespoons of apple cider vinegar
- 1 tablespoon of flat-leaf parsley, chopped
- 1 small clove of garlic
- 2 teaspoons of cilantro, chopped
- ¼ cup of extra virgin olive oil

- ¼ teaspoon of dried dill
- ¼ teaspoon of ground black pepper
- ¼ teaspoon of ground red pepper
- ¼ teaspoon of salt

Procedure:

1. Add the cucumber, parsley, cilantro, garlic, vinegar, red pepper, black pepper, dill and salt to a blender or food processor. Blend until smooth.

2. While processing, slowly add the olive oil. Blend for at least 15 seconds or until the oil is fully absorbed.

3. Pour into a container and store in the refrigerator. Shake well before use.

2. Zucchini Hummus

This is similar to the traditional Middle Eastern version but with a highlight on zucchini, which is low on calories. It can be used as a dip, dressing or spread.

Ingredients:

- 1 ½ zucchinis, chopped
- 3 cloves of garlic
- ¾ cup of sesame seeds
- 1/3 cup of parsley, chopped
- 3 ½ tablespoons of lemon juice
- 1/3 teaspoon of salt

Procedure:

1. Blend seeds in a food processor until it achieves a peanut butter-like consistency (tahini). Set aside.

2. Mince the garlic using the food processor.

3. Add the zucchinis, salt, lemon juice and parsley. Process until crudely chopped.

4. Add the tahini to the processor. Blend until smooth.

3. Italian Herb Tomato Sauce

This sauce is easy to prepare and is much healthier. Tomatoes are also rich in several nutrients such as vitamins A and C, folic acid and lycopene. By making the sauce naturally, you get to take advantage of the nutrients that the tomatoes supply. This sauce will go well with other recipes.

Ingredients:

- 2 ½ cups of fresh tomatoes, chopped
- ¼ cup of sun-dried tomatoes
- 2 ½ teaspoon of dried Italian herbs (e.g. oregano, basil, rosemary and parsley)
- 1 clove of garlic
- ½ celery stalk
- 1/3 teaspoon of salt

Procedure:

1. Soak the sun-dried tomatoes preferably overnight or at for at least 2 hours in water until soft.

2. Mince the herbs, salt, garlic and celery in a food processor.

3. Add the soaked sun-dried tomatoes. Blend well and set aside in a large bowl.

4. Place the chopped fresh tomatoes in food processor and process until chunky and saucy.

5. Add to the sun-dried tomato paste. Stir and mix until fully combined.

4. Soured Coconut Cream

Sour cream is a classic dip found in American and European cuisine. This version utilizes coconut to ensure you stick to your diet. It has a tangy taste plus all the healthy nutrients found in coconuts.

Ingredients:

- ¾ cup of fresh young coconut meat
- 2 teaspoons of lemon juice
- ½ teaspoon of onion powder
- ½ teaspoon of garlic powder
- ½ cup of water

Procedure:

1. Using a blender or food processor, blend all the ingredients until smooth and faintly whipped.

2. Place finished product in a lidded glass jar. Refrigerate.

5. Rawbecue Sauce

This is the raw version of the barbecue sauce and can work well either as a marinade, dip or dressing.

Ingredients:

- 1 dried pepper, soaked
- 1 clove of garlic
- 1 cup of sundried tomatoes, soaked
- 1 cup of fresh tomato, chopped
- 2 tablespoons of yacon syrup
- 2 tablespoons of apple cider vinegar
- 2 teaspoons of chili powder
- 1 teaspoon of nama shoyu
- ½ teaspoon of salt
- ½ cup of soaking water

Procedure:

1. In a blender, place all the ingredients together. Blend until smooth.

2. Store the finished sauce in a glass jar with a lid. Refrigerate.

Breakfast

Considered the most important meal of the day, breakfast is the perfect time for raw food enthusiasts to enjoy meals, from fruits and vegetables to classic breakfast meals with a raw twist. A nutritious meal will allow you to retain your energy throughout the day.

1. Walnut Banana Pancakes

Pancakes are a breakfast favorite, and this recipe allows you to enjoy this childhood favorite and still staying true to the raw food diet. Sadly, this is not the kind of pancake that you can make instantly just by mixing.

Ingredients:

- 6 bananas, sliced
- 2 apples, chopped and cored
- 1 ½ cups of buckwheat
- 1 tablespoon of flax seeds
- 1 cup of sunflower seeds
- 2 tablespoons of coconut flakes
- ½ cup of walnuts, chopped
- 1 ¼ tablespoons of ground cinnamon
- ¼ teaspoon of salt

Procedure:

1. Soak the sunflower seeds and buckwheat overnight or for no less than 6 hours. Rinse well before use.

2. In a coffee grinder or blender, process the flax seeds until it turns into powder. Set aside.

3. In a food processor, blend sunflower seeds and buckwheat until it gets a creamy consistency. Place in a bowl.

4. Process the bananas, apples, salt and cinnamon until smooth. Add to the bowl.

5. Add the walnuts, coconut flakes and flax seeds to the mixture. Mix thoroughly.

6. Prepare ParaFlexx sheets. Shape pancakes by hand. If you have a dehydrator, dehydrate the mixtures for 8 to 12 hours. Otherwise, use an oven until the mixture is dry on the outside but moist inside.

2. Breakfast Tacos with Ruby Raspberry Filling

The romaine lettuce contains antioxidants in its leaves that is said to help battle cancer. It also helps give this recipe a crunchy feel, which is exactly how tacos should be.

Ingredients:

- Breakfast Tacos with Ruby Raspberry Filling
- The romaine lettuce contains antioxidants in its leaves that is said to help battle cancer. It also helps give this recipe a crunchy feel, which is exactly how tacos should be.
- *Ingredients:*
- 4 to 8 romaine leaves
- 1 ruby red grapefruit
- 1 cup of raspberries
- ½ cup of nectarines, diced
- ½ cup of peaches, diced

- 1 teaspoon to 1 tablespoon of agave syrup (optional)

Procedure:

1. Peel the grapefruit and remove the pith using a sharp knife. Then, slice the fruit in half.

2. Place the grapefruit along with the other ingredients (except the leaves) in a mixing bowl. Add agave and toss.

3. Scoop the mix into the romaine leaves.

3. Killer Kasha Porridge

Kasha is a traditional savory dish popular in numerous countries in Eastern Europe and is usually made from buckwheat. This recipe lets you enjoy this dish in its raw form.

Ingredients:

- 2 cups of buckwheat grouts, soaked and sprouted
- 1 cup of apple, chopped
- 2 teaspoons of orange zest
- 1 tablespoon cinnamon
- ½ teaspoon of sea salt

Procedure:

1. Put all the ingredients in a blender or food processor. Blend until it reaches a porridge-like consistency.

2. Scoop into a bowl and serve.

4. Cinnamon Apple Granola

This enjoyable bowl of crunchy granola is another breakfast favorite. You can change it up and use other fruits such as berries, strawberries or bananas.

Ingredients:

- 2 cups of buckwheat
- 2 apples, cored
- 15 dates, pitted
- ¾ cup of almonds
- ½ cup of cashews
- ¾ cup of Brazil nuts
- 1 ½ cups of sunflower seeds
- ½ cup of pumpkin seeds
- ¾ cup of coconut flakes
- 1 tablespoon of ground cinnamon
- 2 tablespoons of hemp protein powder
- 1 tablespoon of maca powder
- 1 teaspoon of vanilla powder
- ½ teaspoon of salt

Procedure:

1. In a bowl, soak almonds, sunflower seeds, pumpkins and buckwheat overnight. Rinse well before use.

2. In a separate bowl, soak Brazil nuts overnight. Rinse well before use.

3. In another bowl, soak cashews overnight. Rinse well before use.

4. In a food processor, process the Brazil nuts until it achieves a medium fine consistency. Add to the bowl of other seeds and nuts along with the cashews.

5. Add the coconut flakes to the bowl.

6. Process the apples, dates, cinnamon, hemp protein powder, salt, vanilla and maca in the food processor until it gets smooth and saucy. Add to the bowl nuts and seeds. Stir thoroughly by hand.

7. Place layers of the mix on ParaFlexx sheets. Place in a dehydrator at 108°F overnight. If you do not have a dehydrator, use an oven and let it bake until the cashews and almonds are crunchy.

5. Creamy Coconut Yogurt

Yogurt is considered a healing food due to the probiotics it contains which helps colonize the digestive tract. The coconut gives this recipe a creamy backdrop for your fruit or garnish of your choice. Coconuts are also rich in healthy fats, helping you stay full during the day.

Ingredients:

- 2 cups of young Thai coconut meat, shredded
- 1 cup of coconut water
- 1 teaspoon of probiotic powder

Procedure:

1. Place the coconut water and coconut meat in a blender. Blend until creamy.

2. Transfer the mix into a container. Add the probiotic powder and stir.

3. Using a piece of cheesecloth or a towel, cover the container and leave for 4-8 hours to sit at room temperature.

4. Serve in a glass or bowl. Store leftovers in the refrigerator.

Note:

You may choose to add other fruits such as bananas or strawberries to give the yogurt more flavors.

Salads

Being a raw foodist, you probably had someone ask you if salads are all you eat. This is part true; salads are an integral part of the raw food diet and are highly nutritious. But contrary to popular belief, salads are not mundane and flavorless. In fact, here are some delectable salad recipes that you may use.

1. Spiked Citrus Curried Quinoa Salad

Sprouted quinoa is a staple in the raw food diet because it is an amazing source of complete protein. This means it has all the amino acids that the body needs. The addition of the spinach, which provides iron, and the orange juice, which is packed in vitamin C that helps the iron be more absorbable, makes this recipe a very healthy meal.

Ingredients:

- 3 cups of sprouted quinoa

- 4 cups of baby spinach
- 2 scallions, chopped
- ½ cup of orange juice
- 2 tablespoons of olive oil
- 1 teaspoon of curry powder
- ½ teaspoon of coriander powder
- ¾ cup of slivered almonds or pine nuts
- ¾ cup of golden raisins
- ¼ cup of red onion, diced

Procedure:

1. In a large bowl, place the quinoa, onion, raisins and almonds or pine nuts. Toss.

2. In another smaller bowl, whisk the olive oil, orange juice, coriander powder and curry powder together. This will become the dressing of the salad.

3. Drizzle the dressing over the larger bowl of quinoa mixture. Toss completely.

4. Serve the mixture over baby spinach and garnish with scallions.

Notes:

Allow the salad to marinate in the dressing for one hour for better taste.

You may use other dried fruits instead of raisins.

If you want a spicier salad, add sliced jalapeños to the mix.

For a tangier flavor, add tangerine chunks.

2. Lettuce Lover's Salad

If you enjoy greens, then you will love this recipe. This particular recipe emphasizes on lettuce but you can easily change up the recipe and use a different vegetable of your liking such as kale, collards, butter leaf, cabbage, red oak and so much more. After all, variety is the spice of life.

Ingredients:

- 2 cups of romaine lettuce, chopped
- 1 cup of Bibb lettuce, chopped
- ½ cup of red-leaf lettuce, torn
- 1/3 cup of celery, sliced
- ¼ cup of carrots, sliced
- 1 cup of arugula, torn
- 1 cup of endive, torn
- 2 tablespoons of olive oil
- 4 teaspoons of coconut vinegar
- ¼ teaspoon of sea salt
- ¼ teaspoon of agave syrup
- 1/8 teaspoon of onion powder
- 1/8 teaspoon of garlic powder
- 1/8 teaspoon of paprika
- ¼ cup of grape tomatoes, sliced

Procedure:

1. Combine the romaine, Bibb and celery lettuce in a bowl. Add the celery, carrots, arugula and endive. Toss to mix.

2. In a separate bowl, whisk the coconut vinegar, olive oil, agave and all the spices to produce the dressing.

3. Drizzle the dressing over the bowl of salad. Toss thoroughly.

4. Garnish with the grape tomatoes and serve.

3. Sprouted Quinoa, Olive and Tomato Salad

This salad goes well on its own or served with the zucchini hummus on the side.

Ingredients:

- 1 cup of quinoa
- ¼ cup of celery, chopped
- ¼ cup of sun dried tomatoes
- 3/8 cup of sun-dried black olives, pitted
- 2 tablespoons of lime juice
- ¼ teaspoon of salt

Procedure:

1. Soak quinoa for 4 hours. Rinse well before use.

2. Soak the sun-dried tomatoes for 2 hours in water until soft.

3. Dice the tomatoes.

4. Toss all the ingredients in a bowl until thoroughly mixed.

4. Sunset Salad

This colorful salad has a bit of sweetness and a bit of spice and can be enjoyed as an afternoon snack to refuel you. It can also be served with a side of guacamole.

Ingredients:

- 2 cups of romaine lettuce, chopped
- 2 cups of pineapple, cubed
- 1 cup of red-leaf lettuce
- 1 small jalapeño, seeded and minced
- ½ red bell pepper, julienned
- ½ cup of fresh pineapple juice
- 2 tablespoons of apple cider vinegar
- 1 tablespoon of fresh chives, diced
- ¼ teaspoon of sweet paprika
- 1/8 teaspoon of ground black pepper
- 1/8 teaspoon of sea salt

Procedure:

1. In a bowl, place the lettuces, bell pepper and pineapple cubes. Toss to mix.

2. In another smaller bowl, combine the pineapple juice and jalapeño pepper. Add the sea salt, black pepper, paprika and apple cider vinegar to make dressing.

3. Toss the salad with the dressing. Chill the finished product before serving.

4. Garnish with fresh chives and serve.

5. Basic Coleslaw Mix

This is a hydrating coleslaw which you can eat on its own or mix with other dishes. You may also add your own touch to it and add other seasonal vegetables in the recipe.

Ingredients:

- 2 carrots, rinsed and trimmed
- 2 cups of green cabbage, roughly chopped
- 1 ¼ cups of red cabbage, roughly chopped

Procedure:

1. Shred the carrots and both cabbages in a food processor subsequently.

2. Toss all the ingredients in a bowl. Combine well.

Main Courses

The main course is an extremely important part of your daily meal plan. Going on a raw food diet does not necessarily mean that your food choices will be boring and repetitive. In fact, here are some healthy raw food main course recipes that you may easily prepare.

1. Veggie Burger Patties

These patties are not only healthy but are also perfect for people with several food allergies.

Ingredients:

- 3 tablespoons of flax seeds
- 3 to 4 stalks of celery stalks
- 2 carrots, chopped
- ½ cup of onions, chopped
- ½ red bell pepper, chopped
- 1 ½ cups of walnuts

- 3/8 cup of sunflower seeds
- 2 tablespoons of hemp seeds
- 1 tablespoon of protein powder
- 2/3 cup of tomatoes, chopped
- ¾ teaspoon of salt

Procedure:

1. Soak the sunflower seeds and walnuts in water overnight or for at least six hours. Rinse well before use.

2. Using a coffee grinder or blender, grind the flax seeds until powder-like.

3. In a food processor, process the tomatoes, carrots, bell peppers, celery, onions, hemp protein and salt into a puree. Place in a bowl.

4. Process the sunflower seeds and walnuts with along with just the right amount of puree to form a paste. Add this to the rest of the puree in the bowl.

5. Add ground flax seeds and hemp seeds. Mix completely by hand.

6. Form the mixture into patties and place on mesh sheets.

7. Let the patties dry using a dehydrator for at least 18 to 24 hours.

2. Petite Beetloaf

This may serve as a main course for two people and the alternative to the usual meat loaf but with healthier, non-meat ingredients. Despite the lack of meat, it contains a hefty dose of protein due to the walnuts and sprouts.

Ingredients:

- ½ cup of cabbage or mung sprouts
- ¼ cup of alfalfa sprouts
- ¼ cup of beets, shredded
- ½ cup of walnuts, soaked for 2 to 4 hours
- 2 tablespoons of celery hearts, chopped
- 2 tablespoons of white or red onion, chopped
- 2 teaspoons of nama shoyu
- Water

Procedure:

1. Using a food processor, grind the walnuts and sprouts along with the nama shoyu.

2. Add the celery, onion and beets to the food processor and process with a bit of water until all the ingredients stick together.

3. Place this mixture in a sheet and shape into a loaf. Dehydrate at 145°F for at least 12 hours.

3. Spiraled Spaghetti Marinara

The marinara is said to be the dish that truly tests the skills of a chef. This version of the famous pasta is perfect for individuals taking on the raw food diet who are lovers of Italian food. In place of the usual flour, zucchini is used to make the noodles.

Ingredients:

- 3 zucchinis
- ½ teaspoon of salt
- ½ cup of soaked sundried tomatoes, soaked water set aside
- 1 cup of tomatoes, chopped
- ½ cup of red bell pepper, chopped
- 1 clove of garlic, minced
- 2 tablespoons of raisins, dates, chopped apples or currants
- 1 tablespoon of olive oil
- 1 ½ teaspoon of any Italian seasoning
- ¼ teaspoon of cayenne pepper powder

Procedure:

1. If you have a spiralizer, use this to turn the zucchinis into long noodles. Otherwise, you may use a vegetable peeler. Stop until you reach the seeds and get rid of the center.

2. Place the zucchini noodles in a bowl and sprinkle the sea salt on top of it. Stir well. Set bowl aside.

3. Using a food processor or blender, process the sundried tomatoes and the water used for soaking together with all the other ingredients except the noodles. Blend until smooth.

4. Gently squeeze the zucchini noodles to completely get rid of any remaining liquid. Mix with the sauce and toss until thoroughly covered. Serve.

4. Tahini Pad Thai

Pad Thai is among the most recognizable Thai dishes available and is starting to become a favorite all over the world. This national dish from Thailand dates back years ago. The raw version of the Pad Thai replaces the peanuts with sesame tahini, removes the fish sauce, egg and leaves out the noodles for a fresher, lighter and healthier meal.

Ingredients:

- 3 zucchinis, medium
- 2 carrots, large
- ¼ cup of sundried tomatoes, soaked in water
- ½ cup of soak water
- 1 tablespoon of tahini
- 2 tablespoons of nama shoyu
- 2 tablespoons of lime juice
- 1 tablespoon of agave syrup
- ½ cup of snow peas
- ½ cup of mung bean sprouts
- ¼ cup of scallions, finely sliced
- 1 clove of garlic, minced
- ½ tablespoon of ginger
- 2 to 4 tablespoons of cilantro, minced
- Lime wedges

Procedure:

1. In a blender, place together the tahini, nama shoyu, sundried tomatoes, ginger, lime juice, agave syrup and garlic and blend until smooth. While blending, slowly pour in the soak water until the mixture turns thick. This will become your pad thai sauce.

2. Turn the carrots and zucchini into noodles using a spiralizer, mandolin or a peeler. You may choose to grate or julienne them alternatively.

3. On a plate, place your noodles, scallions, snow peas and mung bean sprouts. Add the sauce and garnish with the cilantro and lime wedges.

5. Juicy Hues Stir-Dry

This is a vibrant meal, both for the eyes and the mouth, due to the bright colors of the ingredients and their various strong flavors. This main course has the right amount of saltiness, spice and sweetness that you will surely love.

Ingredients:

- 2 cloves of garlic
- 1 red bell pepper, chopped
- 1 orange or yellow bell pepper, chopped
- 1 mango, cubed
- 1 bunch of broccoli, chopped
- 3 scallions, chopped
- 3 tablespoons of nama shoyu
- 2 tablespoons of orange juice
- 1 tablespoon of lime juice
- 1 tablespoon of olive oil
- 1 tablespoon of hot sauce

Procedure:

1. Whisk together the garlic, nama shoyu, lime juice, orange juice, olive oil and hot sauce in a small bowl. Set aside.

2. In a bigger bowl for mixing, toss the mango, bell peppers and broccoli together. Pour the prepared dressing onto the bowl and thoroughly mix until well-coated.

3. Cover the bowl and let it marinate overnight in the refrigerator or for at least 2 hours at room temperature.

4. After letting it marinate, place the bowl to a dehydrator at 110°F for another 2 hours.

5. Garnish using the scallions and serve.

Conclusion

Thank you again for purchasing this book!

I hope this book was able to help you to get a better idea of the raw food diet and provide you with a vast selection of recipes to assure variety in your diet plan.

Change can be overwhelming at times, especially when you are just about to start out. However, if you do not make the changes that are necessary to make your life better, then you will only continue to hold yourself back. If you want to make improvements to your health and whole well-being, the raw food diet may just be the solution you need.

With the raw food diet, you need not rush into anything. You may take things slow and tinker with your routines until you find the right setup for you. While it may be challenging, the rewards that you will reap will all be worth the sacrifice. Let this book be your starting point in progressing towards a raw and healthy lifestyle.

Finally, if you enjoyed this book, please take the time to share your thoughts and post a positive review on Amazon. It'd be greatly appreciated!

In addition, please remember to check out our Facebook page in order to find other resources and upcoming promotions:

https://www.facebook.com/joypublishing

With sincere thanks,

Emma Rose

Preview of 'Clean Eating Guide'
Lose Weight Quickly, Achieve Optimal Health and Feel Energized with Clean Eating for Busy Families and Clean Eating Recipes

Chapter 1
What is Clean Eating?

You have probably come across the term 'clean eating' but you are still not familiar about its exact meaning. This is being used by people who work in the health and fitness industry such as personal trainers ad dietitians. People who are health conscious and workout fanatic also often use this word. Does it have something to do with cleaning the food before eating or cooking? Or maybe it has something to do with the kind of food that you eat.

The loose definition of clean eating is eating food in its most natural state. These days, people are starting to pay more attention to the kinds of food that they eat and how these foods are made. They take note of the food's ingredients and make sure that the food product only contains all natural ingredients.

The term clean eating first came out in the 1990s. Today, it is still being used by health conscious individuals from different backgrounds and culture to refer to the kind of all natural diet that they have. The definition of clean eating can vary from person to person. Some define clean eating as eating mostly fruits and vegetables while others define it as not eating anything artificial. You will find out more about these things as you read this book.

What Clean Eating is not?

If you think clean eating is another diet program, like the South Beach diet or Paleo diet, you are wrong because clean eating is a way of life. It also does not follow any strict rules about what food group to eat and not to eat, how many calories you should consume in a meal, and so on. This is the most basic way of healthy eating that promotes weight loss and boost energy. Everybody can do this, even those who are not trying to lose weight.

Clean eating will not make you feel deprived or frustrated because it is so easy to follow. You do not even need to have a really strong determination because it is all a matter of choosing natural over artificial.

Is there such a thing as 'dirty' eating?

You are probably wondering if there is such a thing as 'dirty' eating or the opposite of clean eating. Clean eating does not literally mean eating foods that have less dirt. It means that you are choosing the best and healthiest food choices from different food groups in their most natural state. 'Dirty' eating is not the opposite of clean eating because there is no such thing as eating dirty. The opposite of clean eating is choosing the wrong food to eat and eating junk foods and processed foods that leave toxins in your body.

Clean eating also looks at the source of food. It should not come from large commercial manufacturers that use machines to process food. The foods that clean eaters usually use come from small farms that do not use chemicals and undergo processes. This is why clean eating is often associated with organic eating.

Check *out the rest of 'Clean Eating Guide' on Amazon*

Or go to: http://www.amazon.com/dp/B00L5FN8RQ/

Detox Diet Guide

Lose Weight Quickly, Achieve Optimal Health and Feel Energized Through the 10 Day Detox

Emma Rose

Table of Contents

Introduction

I want to thank you and congratulate you for purchasing the book, *"Detox Diet Guide: Lose Weight Quickly, Achieve Optimal Health and Feel Energized Through the 10 Day Detox"*.

This book contains proven steps and strategies on how to not just simply flush out toxic substances from our bodies, but to also enhance the way our bodies naturally flush out those toxins.

It also contains other important information such as the most common toxins that are found in the environment that we unknowingly consume, the many ways our bodies naturally detoxify themselves, the things one must and must not do within the ten days of the detox diet, detoxification recipes that can be easily prepared, and some important reminders that must be taken before, during, and after the detox diet.

Thanks again for purchasing this book. I hope you enjoy it! Please take some time to stop by and LIKE our Facebook page:

https://www.facebook.com/joypublishing

With gratitude,

Emma Rose

Chapter 1: Toxins and the Body

As the human body does its usual processes, some things need to be expelled. These are usually waste products made as a result of filtering out substances not needed by the body. There is a reason for the so-called "calls of nature" – which are peeing and releasing excrement.

But sometimes, those unwanted substances can build up in the organs and the bodily systems that comprise them. If there are too much of those substances, they will cause all sorts of harm to the overall bodily functions that can lead to various ailments.

The Top 10 List of Most Common Toxins

Human civilization evolves as a result of the desire of the people to live more comfortably and conveniently. But in the process of that evolution, it has unknowingly unleashed a cavalcade of impurities that do not just pollute the environment, but also the human body. Despite the many efforts by several government agencies and private individuals to thwart the sources of those impurities, there are traces of those impurities that still linger around. Those traces remain in the air, in the soil, in several bodies of water – and eventually, in the foods that humanity consumes.

According to Dr. Joseph Mercola, a well-known personality in the US wellness movement and owner and founder of Mercola.com (one of the most-trusted health websites), the ten most common toxic substances that are still prevalent in the environment to this day are the following:

1. Polychlorinated biphenyls, or PCBs, were commonly dumped by factories into nearby bodies of water. Due to their toxicity, PCBs were banned decades ago. However, traces of PCBs can still be found in those bodies of water since the toxic substances do not break down easily even after all those years. Fish that swim in those bodies of water still consume PCBs

unknowingly. As people still eat those fish, they will also ingest PCBs that will contribute to ailments such as cancer and brain defects in newborn babies.

2. Pesticides, while they do kill pests as their name says, are the major contributors of cancer. As farms still use synthetic pesticides such as weed killers, fungi killers, and insect killers; residues of those pesticides still remain in as much as 50 to 90 percent of US farm produce. Furthermore, there are bug sprays used to kill cockroaches and other unwanted insects in homes. Those bug sprays also contain the same carcinogenic substances as farm-focused pesticides. Besides cancer, pesticides also cause Parkinson's disease, miscarriage, nerve damage, birth defects, and getting in the way of nutrient absorption.

3. Fungal toxins not just come in the form of poisonous mushrooms. The most common of those fungal toxins is mould. Mould thrives in moist places such as bathrooms and kitchens; and can even sustain in vulnerable foods such as peanuts, wheat, and corn. One in three people are allergic to this fungal toxin. If left unchecked, mould causes cancer, heart disease, asthma, multiple sclerosis, and diabetes.

4. Phthalates are commonly found in plastic products and are responsible for softening them, making them easier to mold. They can seep into foodstuffs and drinks that are placed inside plastic food containers and plastic bottles. The result of ingesting too much phthalates is hormonal imbalance, since the substances resemble naturally-produced hormones. In children, phthalates can stunt their growth.

5. Volatile organic compounds, or VOCs, are commonly found in several household products such as air fresheners, cleaning fluids, mothballs, and varnishes. VOCs aid in air pollution and cause several sicknesses such as cancer, irritation of eyes and lungs, headaches, dizziness, and impaired memory.

6. Dioxins are some of the pollutants that are produced when something is burned, especially in massive quantities. As they

are released into the air, humans not just breathe in the dioxins. Livestock can also inhale those toxins and settle in their fats even after they are brought to the slaughterhouse to be made into meat. Dioxins cause cancer, stunted growth, reproductive system impairments, skin disorders such as acne, and slight damage to the liver.

7. Asbestos was a popular insulation material, but it was banned in the seventies due to its carcinogenic effects. Traces of asbestos can still be found in old homes that did not have their insulations replaced. Besides cancer, asbestos causes scarring on the lung tissue.

8. Toxic heavy metals such as lead, arsenic, and mercury can still be found in various objects such as cheaply-made toys, preserved wood, antiperspirants, and building materials. Once those metals are inhaled or ingested, they can cause cancer, brain and nerve disorders such as Alzheimer's disease, nausea, lesser amounts of red and white blood cells, and abnormal heartbeats.

9. Chloroform is a common chemical that is used to make other chemicals. It is prevalent in the air, in water, and in food. It can cause cancer, infertility, birth defects, headaches, dizziness, and damage to the liver and kidneys.

10. Chlorine is commonly found in water as it is used to purify it. Whether from the typical drinking water or from a swimming pool, too much of chlorine will cause all sorts of respiratory problems such as sore throat, accumulation of fluid in the lungs, and asthma.

Based on this list, many of those toxins in the environment are brought about by humanity's modern lifestyles. Before they do undue harm to the body, especially the dreaded cancer, they must be flushed out promptly.

Other Sources of Toxins

Besides the ten most common toxic substances, there are also other toxins that can be found in almost everything in the modern world. It is inevitable that one must intake those toxins unknowingly, one way or the other.

The two most popular vices, which are smoking and drinking, are the other major reasons for the body's toxicity. Both alcohol and nicotine have been proven many times by the scientific community to be not just toxic, but also addicting. Those two substances also alter the brain's functions. Other toxic substances include caffeine, empty sugars, and saturated fats. The latter two are especially notorious for being fat fodder since they cannot be processed into needed energy.

Many cosmetics today also contain toxic substances such as VOCs that can be absorbed into the skin. Some cosmetics producers have already taken steps in ridding their beauty products of those toxins.

Taking too many medications all at once can also cause the body to be laced with toxins, since they are not properly eliminated from the body. If the body feels too taxed from a cornucopia of meds, a consultation with the doctor will help.

There are also naturally-occurring toxins that are used by certain plants and animals as defense mechanisms against invaders. Snakes and jellyfish have highly deadly toxins and should not be consumed as food. A Japanese dish called *fugu* uses a type of blowfish that releases toxins which will certainly kill someone who eats an improperly-prepared version of the dish.

Processed foods, especially canned goods, are also a major source of toxins. While those foods contain preservatives that prolong their shelf lives, they unknowingly unleash a world of hurt on one who voraciously eats these. Needless to say, one must balance those foods out with naturally-grown foods.

Chapter 2: Why Must We Detoxify?

Detoxification is not just the simple flushing out of unwanted substances when the body cannot handle expelling them on its own. It is also the purging of impure thoughts in the mind that cause all sorts of decisions to inhale and ingest several toxins, whether knowingly or unknowingly, into the body. To ensure that an individual is rightfully clean in both body and mind, all sorts of unwanted things must be eliminated, especially in the detox diet.

The Body Does It Own Job...

The excretory system does its job of purging waste substances from the body via its two major processes: urination and release of excrement. Urination is obviously handled by the urinary system, while the release of excrement is handled by the lower parts of the digestive system.

The urinary system's main actor is the kidneys. The kidneys filter unwanted stuff such as ammonia, urea, uric acid, and excess salt and water from the blood as well as other bodily fluids. Those unwanted stuff then get to the bladder, which acts as a temporary storage. If the bladder gets full, the stuff gets expelled out of the urethra in the form of urine. Ammonia is a byproduct of the breakdown and usage of protein for the body's energy, while urea and uric acid are less toxic substances that result from the breakdown of ammonia.

The lower parts of the digestive system consist of the liver, the intestines, and the colon. The liver does its job of breaking down foreign substances so that the kidneys can have an easier job filtering them out as urine. The intestines and the colon facilitate the expelling of solid waste substances in the form of feces. The colon, in particular, absorbs trace minerals such as potassium and sends them to the bloodstream before they are included as feces that will be expelled by pooping.

Another natural detoxifier found in the human body is the lymphatic system. The lymphatic system contains lymph nodes that are scattered throughout the body but are interconnected. Those nodes provide the body with immunity, complementing the immune system, by filtering out unwelcome invaders such as bacteria, viruses, old red blood cells, and other toxic substances.

Other parts of the excretory system consist of the lungs and skin. The lungs expel excess water and carbon dioxide when someone breathes out. The skin kicks out excess water, salt, uric acid, and excess trace minerals in the form of sweat.

...But It Is Not Enough in the Modern Age

However, as demonstrated in the previous chapter, there are far too many substances that are deemed toxic in the wrong amounts. With humanity's modern lifestyles, the body does not know what to make of the increasing number of unwelcome invaders in its insides. These usually never get flushed out as urine and feces, but instead accumulate in the body fat.

As the invaders multiply and never get flushed out, they get in the way of the body's usual processes and will cause several problems such as depleted energy levels, unnatural weight gain, and various diseases that target the major body systems.

Another thing that is not helping the body in its natural detoxification process is the busy and hectic schedules people normally have. Because those people have no time to perform even mundane healthy tasks such as drinking adequate water, the body never gets its supply of natural detox assistants. Couple the lack of those assistants with stress and it will be a recipe for disaster.

Therefore, it is important that in this world of toxicity, people must amplify their bodily defenses against all sorts of foreign toxic substances by enhancing the many components of the excretory system such as the kidneys, the liver, the intestines, and the colon. With the contaminants out of the way, the body's natural healing processes also get their groove back. As the major organ systems work hand-in-hand, the benefits that are felt in one particular system will spread towards the other systems.

In short, steeling the body and its functions, especially the excretory functions, is one of the first lines of defense against toxin-induced sicknesses. There will be a marked loss in weight, since the excessive fats as well as the toxins they contain are properly expelled. There will also be renewed liveliness since the bodily functions that have something to do with the intake and processing of energy sources are no longer clogged by invasive toxins.

Why the Mind Is Also Important in Detoxification

The decisions a person makes, no matter how small they are, can contribute to huge consequences. For example, if one decides to commute to a bar, he or she gets all sorts of toxins in the process – airborne impurities from urban roads, food additives from the snacks he or she eats while commuting, nicotine and other chemicals from tobacco smoke generated by smokers inside and outside the bar, and alcohol from the hard drinks he or she consumes while in the bar.

Therefore, it is important that a person must think thoroughly and deeply before settling on a decision that will make him or her take in all those unwanted toxins along the way. Yes, this may turn him or her into a control freak, but there are also decisions that will endow him or her with long-term benefits. Remember, detoxification starts in the mind. The decisions that lead to the unknowing intake of toxins must be sorted out and eliminated from the usual routines first.

Chapter 3: The Crucial Ten Days

There are several forms of detoxification, and they more often than not involve ingesting special liquids and solids, cleansing the colon, foot baths and foot pads, spas and saunas, and fasting. But they also cost money, are always focused on the short-term effects, and may not deliver the detoxification results one desires. The best form of the detox diet must involve getting rid of major sources of toxins, ingesting more of the substances that will greatly assist the body's natural detoxification processes, never integrating any form of starvation or elimination of a major food group from the diet, and clearing the mind of impure thoughts that lead to impure actions. This way, the diet will grant long-term effects of well-being. As a beneficial consequence, this diet will cost little to no money, except for the money to be spent on detoxifying foods and drinks.

The ten days this detox diet contains are important to ensure natural weight loss and general well-being. And even after the diet period ends, some good habits contained in this diet, particularly the continued eating of healthy foods, must still be kept. This is to ensure that the person undergoing this diet will transition into a healthy lifestyle.

Preparing for the Diet

One important thing to do when undergoing this diet, or any other diet for that matter, is to not rush in immediately. A crash diet will have nasty consequences such as abrupt changing of body patterns that lead to all sorts of ailments as well as retention of the weight one lost during the diet routine. Therefore, one must start slow and transition into the diet carefully.

Not rushing in also applies to the chewing of food. The body needs some time to digest the food. Never treat the ten days of the diet like some kind of work deadline.

The usual vice-based sources of toxins, which are tobacco and alcohol, must be eliminated first. While dealing with the withdrawal effects of both of those substances may be difficult, timely help from a doctor who has a specialization in several types of addictions and substance abuse will lessen the difficulty.

In the three days before the actual start of the diet, rid the pantry and fridge of tempting foodstuffs that are loaded with empty calories. These include sweets and most forms of processed foods and fast food. At the same time, steadily increase the intake of fruits and vegetables – *especially organic ones*. As much as possible, turn the veggies into freshly-prepared salads and/or lightly steam them. As for the fruits, eat them raw and/or turn them into natural juices.

Since pesticide residue in fruits and vegetables is inevitable, the use of fruit and vegetable washes must be prioritized.

The intake of caffeine must be slowly and surely reduced to prevent withdrawal symptoms such as headaches. Switching to decaf coffee and low-caffeine teas such as green tea will help, as is the trick of diluting regular coffee and tea in huge amounts of water.

And speaking of water, the time-tested advice of eight to ten glasses of water a day will especially help the detox diet become successful. Drink it throughout the ten days of the diet.

Aromatherapy using essential oils is helpful, as this therapy helps to calm the mind in order for it to prepare for the rigors of the critical ten days.

Finally, before embarking on the detox diet itself, please consult a registered dietician who can recommend the detoxifying foods to be eaten based on your genetic makeup. Furthermore, *do not stop* taking prescribed medicine, as discontinuing medications can have devastating effects on the body. Diets are not meant to be one-man shows, especially if the individual still has to learn much about the intricacies of diet programs like this.

Eat and Drink Them

With the transition phase over, it is time to actually start the detox diet. Here is a comprehensive list of foods and drinks that must be ingested during the ten crucial days of the diet.

1. Organic fruits and vegetables are the main focus of the detox diet. It does not matter what the size or type of fruit or vegetable one will be consuming – as long as it is free of pesticides and synthetic fertilizers and is grown using age-old farming techniques, it certainly counts. Eat a good variety of fruits and vegetables to round out all the necessary nutrients.

2. Brown rice is much healthier compared to the typical white rice. As white rice is a result of the milling process, brown rice retains some nutrients that are usually lost during milling. This type of rice is also a rich source of fiber, which will aid in flushing the toxins out via the intestines and the colon.

3. Herbs are permissible, since they are also plants. Use them to flavor the dishes as well as utilize them for aromatherapy. Herbal teas are also a-OK, since they do not contain caffeine at all. As with fruits and vegetables, herbs must not have traces of anything toxic.

4. Whole-grain products, much like brown rice, do not undergo the nutrient-losing milling process. They are also rich sources of fiber. Whole-grain products include whole wheat bread, bran, and rolled oats.

5. Seaweeds such as kelp and *nori* wrappers used for sushi are also plant-based. They can also be consumed the same way as typical veggies do.

6. Beans such as green peas, chick peas, lentils, kidney beans, and black beans are permitted.

7. One can go nuts with nuts and seeds. Allowable things include almonds, cashews, walnuts, watermelon seeds, pumpkin

seeds, sunflower seeds, and sesame seeds. As a general rule, pick only raw, unsalted nuts and seeds.

8. Coconuts, while they are not actually nuts, are also allowed. There are several coconut-based consumables such as coconut water and coconut oil. One can also eat fresh coconut meat straight from the source.

9. Plant-based oils are encouraged. Olive oil, especially the extra virgin kind, is highly recommended.

10. Round out the protein-based nutrition with plant-based protein sources such as soy. Soy milk and tofu are easily-acquired sources of plant-based protein.

11. All sorts of edible mushrooms are permitted. Portobello and shiitake mushrooms can act as good substitutes for meat.

12. Natural sweeteners such as raw honey and natural maple syrup are permitted.

13. Besides herbs, other natural condiments that are tolerable include apple cider vinegar, sea salt, and mustard.

14. If there is still a desire to eat meat and get adequate protein, go with lean meats such as fish and organic chicken. Eggs are also on the list, as long as they are organic.

Never Eat and Drink Them

Meanwhile, these are the foods and drinks to avoid during the detox diet phase.

1. In general, non-lean types of red meat are off-limits. Canned meat is especially forbidden.

2. All forms of processed foods containing all sorts of additives and preservatives are out of the question. On a related note, artificial sweeteners and processed condiments are also out.

3. Typical white sugar and brown sugar are verboten, as well as high-fructose syrups.

4. Corn must be avoided as it is acid-forming. The acid in question is uric acid. Furthermore, the corn kernels that are indigestible will make bathroom breaks more excruciating.

5. While nuts are OK, peanuts and peanut butter are usually excluded.

6. Milk is normally not allowed, but half a cup of yogurt containing good bacteria per day is an exception to that.

7. Caffeine is another typical forbidden substance.

8. Shortening and margarine are inadmissible.

9. While fish is OK, other seafoods are not.

Other Cleansing Procedures

There are many variations of the detox diet, but the one being presented in this book will not involve complicated doohickeys and specialized food and drinks to amplify the detoxification effect. Here are some things one can also do during the ten days of the diet.

With all the conveniences of Internet-based connectivity, sometimes too much is too much. Dedicate one of the ten days, or even all ten days, to a temporary break from technology. Put away the smartphone or tablet, avoid touching the computer, and never be tempted to go online just about anywhere. Take the time off from technology to visit someplace serene, like a retreat house. This technology break will clear the mind of all sorts of burdening thoughts that may poison one's thinking the same way that bodily toxins do.

Take some time off to scrape the tongue. Tongue scraping is a practice in ayurvedic medicine, or ancient Hindu medicine, where all the impurities built up on the tongue are removed. Tongue scrapers can be bought for cheap at drug store.

Try to write all the stored thoughts and feelings, even negative ones, into a diary or notebook. Releasing all the stored strong emotions to a diary or notebook has a cathartic effect, since keeping those emotions locked away will eventually take the toll on one's health.

Another mind-cleansing procedure one can do during the ten days is meditation. Meditation also helps clear the mind of toxic thoughts that lead to stress, which then slows down the liver's detoxification process. Yoga is especially helpful as a meditation tool. You may also augment your meditation by doing deep breathing exercises or visualizing relaxing images such as watching the sunset at the beach.

Get enough dosages of vitamin C. While the vitamin is better known for boosting immunity, it also helps the body with the production of glutathione. Glutathione may be better known as a skin rejuvenating agent, but it also exists in the liver as a detoxification aid. Citrus fruits are the best-known sources of vitamin C.

Enhance blood circulation, since poor blood circulation will hamper the flushing out of impurities from the blood. Exercise is a guaranteed way to get that blood pumping.

Keep in mind that not all bacteria are bad. Good bacteria mostly reside in the intestines, aiding in digestion and preventing bad bacteria from releasing toxins that can be deployed in the bloodstream. Help the good bacteria by taking probiotic drinks.

Chapter 4: Detoxification Recipes

Breakfast Recipes

Gut-Busting Oatmeal Bowl

Ingredients:

- 1-2 cups oatmeal

- 1-2 cups water or nut milk

- A mixture of fresh berries and fresh fruits, all sliced

Procedure:

1. Prepare the oatmeal as indicated in the packaging.

2. While hot, pour the berries and fruits onto the prepared oatmeal, and mix.

Berry Blast Smoothie

Ingredients:

- 1-2 cups mixed fresh berries
- 1-2 cups protein powder
- 1-2 cups ice cubes

Procedure:

1. Throw all the ingredients into a blender, and hit puree.
2. Serve the smoothie in a tall glass.

Lunch Recipes

Veggie Cavalcade Salad with Tofu

Ingredients:

- 6-8 pieces of any whole vegetable (for greens, an amount of at least five leaves equals one whole piece)

- 1-2 pieces tofu, diced

- 4-5 teaspoons extra virgin olive oil

- 2 teaspoons fresh lemon juice

- 1 teaspoon freshly-chopped herbs of choice

Procedure:

1. Fry the tofu in 2-3 teaspoons olive oil until slightly browned. Set aside.

2. Slice and/or dice the vegetables into reasonably-sized pieces. Leave the greens untouched.

3. Pour all the vegetables and the tofu into a bowl. Mix completely.

4. Combine 2 teaspoons olive oil, the lemon juice, and the herbs to make the dressing.

5. Pour the dressing all over the salad. Mix completely.

Special Omelet Rice

Ingredients:

- 3-5 organic eggs
- Fresh or dried herbs (any variety), to taste
- 2-3 teaspoons extra virgin olive oil
- 1-2 cups cooked brown rice

Procedure:

1. Beat the eggs into a scramble while adding the herbs.
2. Pour the olive oil into a heated pan. Wait until the oil is hot.
3. Pour the egg and herb mixture until the omelet is formed. Turn over to ensure proper cooking.
4. Once the omelet is out of the pan, place the brown rice inside it. Make sure the omelet wraps around the rice.
5. Serve hot with mustard.

Dinner Recipes

The Steamed Medley

Ingredients:

- 1 slice salmon

- 5-10 pieces broccoli and asparagus (can be of any combination)

- 1/4 cup fresh lemon juice

- Fresh or dried herbs (any variety), to taste

Procedure:

1. In a steamer or a rice cooker with a steaming basket, arrange the salmon slice and the broccoli and asparagus pieces so that the steam will be evenly distributed.

2. Sprinkle the salmon and the vegetables with the lemon juice and fresh herbs.

3. Begin steaming the salmon and the vegetables. Seven to ten minutes is enough for the lemon and the herbs to seep into the steamed content.

4. Serve hot.

Glorified Bunch of Small Potatoes

Ingredients:

- 6 ounces small potatoes

- 4 tablespoons extra virgin olive oil

- Any natural condiment of choice

Procedure:

1. Gently simmer the potatoes in water for 5-10 minutes. Drain them off afterwards. Retain the peels beforehand.

2. Heat the olive oil in a roasting tin, but not to burning levels.

3. Roast every side of the potatoes until crisp and golden brown. This will take at most 45 minutes.

4. Serve hot with the condiment of choice.

Snack and Drink Recipes

Veggie Brown Rice Sushi

Ingredients:

- 1 cup cooked brown rice
- 1 *nori* wrapper
- Any sliced or diced vegetable that can fit inside the sushi

Procedure:

1. Mold the brown rice into any shape, whether in a tube form or rolled into a ball. The important thing is that the vegetable must fit inside the sushi.

2. Wrap the *nori* wrapper around the formed brown rice.

3. Repeat steps 1 and 2 for any remaining amounts of vegetables, brown rice, and the *nori* wrapper.

Stretched Herbal Iced Tea

Ingredients:

- 1 bag herbal tea (any kind)
- 1 citrus fruit of choice (e.g. lemon or orange)
- 1 cup briskly-boiled water
- 2-3 cups lukewarm water
- Several ice cubes
- Honey, to taste

Procedure:

1. Depending on the strength of the resultant tea, submerge one teabag into briskly-boiled water.

2. Meanwhile, cut the citrus fruit of choice into slices that can be fit inside a glass.

3. Place the fruit slices into a tall glass that can accommodate at least five cups.

4. Carefully pour both the brewed tea and the lukewarm water into the tall glass at a distance of at least 12 inches from the glass. This is where the "stretched" part comes from, and one must avoid spills during the stretching process.

5. Add some dollops of honey based on the preferred amount of sweetness.

6. Finally, add the ice cubes.

Fruity Shaved Ice

Ingredients:

- 1-2 cups shaved ice

- 1/2-1 cup natural unsweetened fruit juice of any kind

Procedure:

1. Place the shaved ice in either a wide glass or a bowl.

2. Pour the unsweetened fruit juice on top of the shaved ice, and enjoy.

Note: One can replace shaved ice with shaved or crushed frozen fruit.

Chapter 5: Some Friendly Reminders

As with every other diet program on the planet, care, precise planning, patience, and perseverance must be taken to heart when undergoing the detoxification diet. Even in a short period like ten days, many things will happen. To ensure that the detox diet will become a success that will beget many more successes in the realm of the healthy lifestyle, keep the following friendly reminders in mind.

Do Not Starve

Other detox diets recommend taking only the formulas they sell themselves. Indeed, they may contain needed plant-based nourishment needed for detoxification, but the makers of those diets often forget that an imbalanced diet that is lacking in calories will prove detrimental to the body. Not only will the energy levels be depleted, but the metabolism process will also be slowed down. One unpleasant aftereffect is the tendency to eat more, especially unhealthy foods, once the diet period is over. This will make natural weight loss almost unachievable. Even worse, the lack of micronutrients in these other detox diets will lead to malnutrition that is based on micronutrient deficiency, which opens yet another floodgate of diseases. Other nasty effects of other detox crash diets include muscle degeneration, since the muscles have no source of energy to turn to, and an imbalance in blood sugar levels.

Hence, this detox diet espouses the idea that *forced starvation is absolutely prohibited.* Just eat the recommended foods at will and in good, moderated amounts.

Expect to Pee (and Poop and Sweat) a Lot

Since the detox diet enhances the body's natural detox functions, expect one undergoing the diet to pee a lot. Water, in particular, helps in flushing out toxins.

Excessive peeing not just happens when the detox diet goes overboard. Excessive sweating also happens, as well as the resultant excrement being too liquid and nasty-smelling. Peeing, pooping, and sweating too much can lead to dehydration if the amount of fluids being taken is not immediately replenished.

Dehydration is not just the depletion of the body's water, but is also the disrupted balance of fluids and electrolytes that can lead to ailments such as gastrointestinal distress, headaches, fatigue, irritability, skin irritations, circulatory problems, kidney failure, and heat stroke. Death also awaits one who is severely dehydrated.

To counteract dehydration, do not depend on fluids and fluids alone, unlike what some detox diets emphasize. Be well-balanced in both solids and liquids to avoid lost hours as a result of abnormally frequent trips to the bathroom.

Want a Colonic? No Thanks

Another form of the detox therapy involves cleansing the colon and intestines of toxins that may be released into the bloodstream. However, as demonstrated in the third chapter, there are beneficial bacteria that reside in the colon and intestines. If those bacteria are flushed out, the normal digestive process will be hampered, and the bad bacteria will have a good time releasing more toxins since their rivals are gone. The flushing out of good bacteria also results from the detox diet going beyond the recommended ten days.

Another bad effect of colon cleansing is dehydration, for the same reasons demonstrated in the previous section. Trace minerals such as potassium are also lost during the cleansing process, which contributes to dehydration. Other side effects of colon cleansing include nausea and vomiting.

Diet as an End to the Means, Not a Means to the End

People who want the figures of their dreams often forget that dieting is not really meant to immediately shed unwanted pounds. Dieting is truly meant for improved nourishment and nutrition. The notions of shedding that slab or beer belly in preparation for an event like showing off in a bikini should be disposed of. A proper mindset must be established first when doing the detox diet or any other diet for that matter.

As stated before, the detox diet being demonstrated in this book should be a transitional phase to a healthier lifestyle. Thinking in the long term when dieting is certainly better than thinking in the short term. One should remember that dieting must be an end to unhealthy habits and not a means to end that "awful" figure.

Conclusion

Thank you again for purchasing *"Detox Diet Guide: Lose Weight Quickly, Achieve Optimal Health and Feel Energized Through the 10 Day Detox"*!

I hope this book was able to help you to understand the ins and outs of the detox diet and why it is important to achieve a major change in only a short time.

Are you ready for the change? Tony Robbins says in order to create effective change, you need to start by being disgusted with where you are at. Are you disgusted with your health or body? Is it an ABSOLUTE MUST to change...not another moment? You need to feel the pain of where you are at to get the urgency to change and manifest the momentum to take action.

The next step is to consult your doctor or dietician before embarking on such a diet. And once you are given the final OK, you can then consult various more detoxification recipes based on the comprehensive list of allowable foods and drinks in this book. The recipes given in this book is just a starting point.

Finally, if you enjoyed this book, please take the time to share your thoughts and post a review on Amazon. It would be greatly appreciated!

I would love for you to share your experiences, stories and encouragements with me. My email address is

emmarosekindle@gmail.com

In addition, please remember to check out our Facebook page in order to find other resources and upcoming promotions:

https://www.facebook.com/joypublishing

With sincere thanks,

Emma Rose

Preview Of "Paleo Free Diet Guide for Beginners: Over 50 Paleo Free Diet Recipes for Fast Weight Loss and Optimal Health"

Introduction

I want to thank you and congratulate you for purchasing the book, *"Paleo Free Diet Guide for Beginners: Over 50 Paleo Free Diet Recipes for Optimal Health and Fast Weight Loss"*.

This book contains everything you might need to know when it comes to getting started with the Paleo diet. It is provided in an easily digestible format that allows you to better absorb the information. There are no complicated explanations about how it works! You'll be given what you need straight up so you won't have to waste time trying to understand exactly what the diet is. Whether it's for your overall good health or to lose a few pounds, Paleo can certainly help you with it. To help you get started, we'll do the same and start you off with 50 of the best Paleo recipes that you can slowly but surely shift your everyday menu to.

It's never easy changing a diet. I often fall into self pity when I can no longer have the foods I enjoy. Either I feel sorry for myself or I get rebellious and binge and anything and everything. I always knew the value of eating healthy. I could just never bring myself to do it. It wasn't until I had a miscarriage that I got serious about my health. I have made drastic changes that others just don't understand. But the pay off is the weight I've lost and the better health I'm experiencing.

My hope for you is not to be on another "diet." This isn't a restriction diet like Atkins. The goal is to have a lifestyle change. Lifestyle changes are more sustainable and maintain weight loss long term compared to restriction diets. The change is hard to start but worth it when you commit. The trick is to get the momentum to start.

Thanks again for purchasing this book. I hope you enjoy reading it and eating the recipes from it!

With gratitude,

Emma Rose

Chapter 1 – What Is the Paleo Diet?

The Paleo Diet is known by many names such as the cavemen diet, stone age diet and hunter-gatherer diet, to name a few. The concept behind this diet follows that of the Paleolithic era before the development of agriculture. Essentially, you consume the same foods that the cavemen used to eat. The focus is on eating food closest to its natural, unprocessed state. The cavemen would gather their food from any source available whether it was wild animals, berries, vegetables, or fruits. As a result, they were strong, fit, and healthy for thousands of years.

This type of diet is still very young, less than fifty years only, but more in depth researches and studies are being conducted to increase the information and knowledge on this diet. The results of previous studies conducted on the Paleo diet reveal the improvement of health to the people involved. This is attributed to the fact that no processed foods and additives are included. The Paleo Diet is a diet that works with our genetics – before machinery and processing got involved. Foods that were not available during the Paleolithic time such as dairy products, salt, sugar and grains are not included in the preparation of the Paleo diet.

The modern diet predominately consumed in the Western world is full of refined foods, trans fats, salt and sugar. These ingredients are known to indirectly cause diseases such as hypertension, diabetes, strokes, obesity and other heart problems. The list goes on even further with the increase diagnosis of cancer, Parkinson's, Alzheimer's, depression and infertility. "What an extraordinary achievement for a civilization: to have developed the one diet that reliably makes its people sick!" (Michael Pollen, Food Rules: An Eater's Manual, Penguin Books 2009).

Foods included in the Paleo Diet

- Fruit

- Vegetables

- Lean Meat

- Seafood

- Nuts/Seeds

- Healthy Fats (eg. coconut, avocado, nuts and seeds, olive oil, grass fed butter)

Foods NOT included in the Paleo Diet

- Dairy

- Grain

- Processed Food

Why not grain?

You may be surprised to see that grains are not included in the Paleo Diet. We are accustomed to grains being a part of a balanced diet. However, our bodies are not designed to deal with the nutritional components of grains such as gluten, lectin, and phytates.

Gluten is a protein substance found in wheat, barley and rye. Many people are discovering that their bodies are gluten sensitive and are eliminating gluten from their diet. The most extreme case of gluten sensitivity is Celiac Disease. Individuals with this disease can pick up the minutest trace of gluten and react immediately.

Lectin binds to insulin receptors and can also cause leptin resistance.

Phytates cause minerals to become unavailable during digestion.

Why is dairy a problem?

When purchasing milk, you need to be mindful of the source.

Check out the rest of "Paleo Diet Guide for Beginners: Over 50 Paleo Diet Recipes for Fast Weight Loss and Optimal Health" on Amazon.

Or go to: http://amzn.to/1jIJUFX

Check Out My Other Books

Below you'll find some of my other books also available on Amazon and Kindle. Search for these titles on the Amazon website to find them.

Paleo Free Diet Guide for Beginners: Over 50 Paleo Free Recipes for Optimal Health & Fast Weight Loss

Paleo Desserts: Satisfy Your Sweet Tooth With Over 100 Quick & Easy Paleo Dessert Recipes & Paleo Baking Recipes

Raw Food Diet Guide: Lose Weight Quickly, Achieve Optimal Health & Feel Energized with the Raw Food Diet & Raw Food Recipes

Clean Eating Guide: Lose Weight Quickly, Achieve Optimal Health & Feel Energized with Clean Eating For Busy Families & Clean Eating Recipes

Alkaline Diet Guide: Lose Weight Quickly, Achieve Optimal Health & Feel Energized with the Alkaline Diet & Alkaline Recipes

Coconut Flour Recipes for Optimal Health & Quick Weight Loss: Gluten Free Recipes for Celiac Disease, Gluten Sensitivities & Paleo Free Diets

Almond Flour Recipes for Optimal Health & Quick Weight Loss: Gluten Free Recipes for Celiac Disease, Gluten Sensitivities & Paleo Free Diets

Wheat Free Diet for Beginners: Lose Weight Quickly, Achieve Optimal Health & Feel Energized with Gluten Free Recipes for Celiac Disease, Gluten Sensitivities & Paleo Free Diets

Detox Diet Guide: Lose Weight Quickly, Achieve Optimal Health & Feel Energized Through the 10 Day Detox

Sugar Detox Guide for Beginners: Lose Weight Quickly, Achieve Optimal Health, Feel Energized & Eliminate Sugar Cravings Naturally

Ketogenic Diet Guide for Beginners: How to Achieve Rapid Weight Loss, Optimal Health & Unstoppable Energy with Ketogenic Diet Recipes

Anti Inflammatory Diet for Beginners: Lose Weight Fast, Optimize Health, Slow Aging, Fight Inflammation, Conquer Pain & Increase Energy with the Anti Inflammation Diet Recipes

One Last Thing...

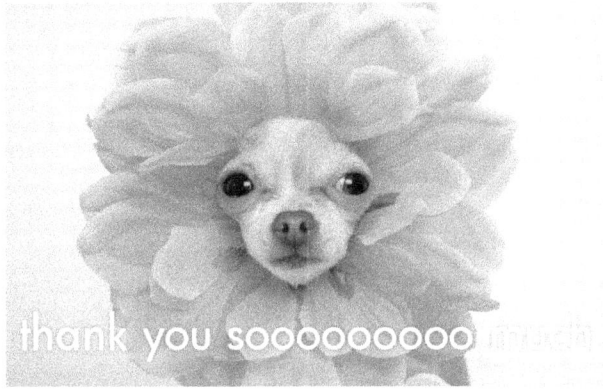

Source: Wikipedia

If you believe that this book is worth sharing, would you please take the time to let others know how it affected your life? If it turns out to make a difference in the lives of others, they will be forever grateful to you, as will I.